I0439935

The Absolutely Essential Guide to Erotic Breast Massage – Special Edition – 5 Books in One!

Michelle Tallia

ISBN-13: 978-1490493534
ISBN-10: 1490493530

Erotic BDSM Books - Your Erotic BDSM Book Publisher
EroticBDSMbooks.com

This book includes 4 free bonus books (making it a $34.75 value!) Your five books are presented in this order:

Other Books by Phil G Include:

The Absolutely Essential Book of BDSM and S&M Rules
Things To Do During 3 Hours of Sex; A Step-by-step Guide
Playtime At The Dom Den; A Step-by-step Guide
The Absolutely Essential Guide to Great BDSM and S&M Sex
The Absolutely Essential Dominant/submissive Playtime Experience
The Absolutely Essential BDSM Sexual Experience
The Ultimate Collection of S&M and BDSM Rules For Female Submissives and Slaves
Master and submissive or slave BDSM Contract
Mistress/slave BDSM Contract
The Funniest BDSM Personal Ads
Have Awesome BDSM Sex
BDSM Master/slave Contract
Spanking Dictionary
BDSM Rules
Bed Arrest, the Punishment for BDSM Enthusiasts

Book 1

100 Great Lines To Put in Your Personal Ad

Introduction

The lines in this book can be combined with other lines you may think of to make your personal ad all it can be. Some lines in the book might need adapting to best suit you and/or your sex.

TAGLINES: Your short "tagline" is a headline that, perhaps along with your picture, can get readers to further explore your ad. Great taglines are like gold and people have paid hundreds of dollars for them! Now however many are on the Internet for you to see and use.

Remember, people love to laugh. A funny tagline is a big plus.

There is a great deal of material in this book to build quality taglines from. You may also want to take a bit of time and do a web search for "best personal ad taglines" for ideas. Chances are others (including those looking at your ad) haven't seen the tagline already, or have forgotten it if they did.

The Lines

A day not in love is a lost opportunity.

My friends know me as spontaneous, spritely, and upbeat.

I am searching for a beautiful person inside and out.

Are you looking for real love and someone special?

I enjoy thought provoking dialogue.

Together let's seek our destiny.

I hope only to fulfill your every desire. Is that too much to ask?

I love making people happy and to see them smile, even if at times it is at my own expense.

I feel the most pleasure when I know I am doing/enduring something to please another.

I'm looking to learn, not just to play....

I'd like to explore hidden fantasies with you.

I want to be taken to that special place and beyond.

I have the financial and emotional capacity to take care of myself.

Unlike perhaps others here I'm not misrepresenting myself. I know the importance of honesty.

I need to be with someone who has a high self esteem, is confident in themselves and who if they have baggage, knows how to deal with it. I love challenges too so if you dare me I won't hesitate to do it.

I love sex. Rough sex, fun sex, emotional sex... I want you to respect me before and after but during is negotiable.

I want to explore my naughty side,

I'm looking for a friend, confidant and lover.

Like me I'd like you to be thoughtful, attractive, and looking to expand yourself as a person.

I have developed intricate pleasure techniques which can slowly arouse and pleasure beyond imagination.

I think I would describe myself, briefly, as quite a sociable person with a good sense of humor who doesn't take herself too seriously...having said that I believe I am also thoughtful and caring and someone who places great value on good friendships and relationships.

I am loyal, compassionate and respectful of people and animals. People describe me as easy going and good natured.

I have got great plans and goals in my life which I want to achieve.

I'm a contemporary yet spiritual soul in search of his charming, compassionate and caring companion to share this journey of life.

Are you looking for someone to grow with and push things further?

I have a wise mind and younger spirit.

I am an easy going, and loyal friend.

I'm looking forward to a fantastic voyage of a relationship.

I am attracted to someone who enjoys learning and growing.

Are you looking for fun, adventure and a challenge? If so I'm your girl.

I'm a passionate person with interests numerous and diverse.

I am trustworthy, affectionate, passionate, loving and non-judgmental. I am happy with myself and my accomplishments.

I want someone kind, loving, honest, communicative and self-aware. Your developed interest in education, hygiene, aesthetics, style and emotional literacy would make life easier for us. I'd like to find someone interested in building a relationship based on an accomplished life and a win/win attitude.

I am looking for someone who can work themselves deep inside my mind and make me fall to my knees.

Are you looking for someone to make you happy...someone that won't just have sex with you but will make love to you?

We all want to achieve heart pounding serenity.

I am looking for something more than just sex and games. Sure sex is a part of it but I also want someone that I can spend time with. I want the total package.

I want someone that I can go out with, talk with, laugh with, and fall in love with.

Outside of our playtime, I'd like to enjoy a harmony that can grow into a loving, trusting relationship. I enjoy the outdoors and staying healthy, going out on the town from time to time and hanging out at home.

My last relationship ended because we grew in different directions.

I am usually lucky and love life. I would like to find someone like that.

I'm a strong, seductive, passionate woman who is established and knows herself.

I'm well educated and well-travelled. I'm gainfully employed and very independent. I enjoy traveling, good food and wine, the theater and sports.

I'm searching for an open minded man with an adventurous soul and sensual heart. A journey in love is the destination. We still have plenty of time but none to waste! A beautiful world is waiting. Let's enjoy while we can!

I'll laugh at your corny jokes.

I'm a writer and voracious reader. I'm smart, and I like smart people.

Physical attraction leads to animal instincts.

I have a strong passion for the exploration and power of touch in all its forms.

I enjoy knowledge, I like to learn new and exciting things.

I am cosmopolitan and highly educated. I am a baby boomer, in good shape and would like an agemate and a partner who understands mutuality. I am interested in developing a long term relationship.

I am interested in meeting someone who is honest, open and enjoys (his)her kink.

I have very many interests and I'm passionate about all of them! I love movies, literature, music, art, theatre, science… and lots of other things.

I am fun, open-minded, spontaneous and down for raunchy action.

The reason openness is important to me is that it shows that someone accepts themselves.

I'm lively and active and have a well developed sense of humor.

I hope to always be me and take advantage of any opportunities and chances whenever they're thrown at me.

I am totally devoted when in love.

I'm a laid-back, drama-free kind of person.

I want to be late to my own funeral.

Physical play is quite enjoyable but chemistry and a connection is more important.

I like to laugh, I like to have fun.

I believe that love is not what we see but what we do.

I won't ignore you or abandon you. I'm not looking for a secondary relationship.

I have a well developed and dominant sexual identity. I am seeking a man who is a smart, uninhibited, challenging partner.

I consider myself a natural leader, an innovator, a creator. I fight for the best and readily take the risks incumbent with leading a fulfilled, enriched life.

I am a strong, confident thinker, with a secure sense of himself (herself).

I consider myself to be a spontaneous, fun loving person. I work hard, play hard, and enjoy life. I'm a very affectionate and passionate. I like to hold hands and believe it or not cuddle. I believe in treating others the way I would like to be treated.

I am looking for someone to grow with spiritually, mentally and physically. I want someone who is not afraid to love and be loved, someone who is affectionate, passionate and good kisser.

I will love you and take good care of you. I am someone who you can trust and believe in, someone who will always want to make you feel happy.

I'm neat and clean both internally and externally.

I want true love and real commitment.

I am looking for something more than just sex and games. There is a balance that is needed since none of us can live in a purely sexual world. Sure sex is an important part of it all but I also want someone that I can spend time with. I want the total package. I want someone I can go out with, talk with, laugh with, and fall in love with.

I want something that will naturally grow and evolve into its own very beautiful story.

I enjoy a great number of things and am very open to experimentation.

I'm interested in your fantasies.

I want to touch your body, your soul, your life.

I still believe that fairytales can come true, it can happen to us...

I live a healthy lifestyle. I am seeking the same.

I am brimming with sexual desire.

I will be looking forward to hear from you and Your wish will always be done...

I am looking for a partner - but I am happy to form a friendship.

Living on earth is expensive...but it does include free trips around the sun.

I eat healthy and workout regularly.

I am an educated, intelligent professional with eclectic tastes in most everything: art, music, food, people, entertainment and travel.

I'm looking for a non-smoker to share my life with in all ways, a friend and companion to travel with, commiserate over bad days and rejoice over good days; a lover and confidant.

Educated, professional and kinky.

I have class and style. I know the value of dressing to impress.

I would love to be able to say "I've finally found you."

I believe that we all have the ability to create or change anything.

I consider myself to be a sharp, crafty, inventive, fun, strong woman who enjoys life more when she's in a relationship.

I'm looking for a like minded man to chat, debate and play with.

I'm not a just fantasist wasting your time.

I am people biased not gender biased.

I am family-oriented and have family values.

I possess confidence but take pride in not being arrogant. I'm persistent but respectful. I have intelligence and charm.

I don't like negative people. We're here to live life not fear it.

I have learned in life that the smallest good deed is better than the grandest good intention. I have high hopes for us.

I am a sharp, crafty, inventive, fun woman who doesn't hate men or hate anyone for that matter.

I enjoy life so much more when I'm in a relationship.

What you are like OUT of bed makes you more desirable for me to want you to take me there.

I like to please as much as be pleased.

I want to discover and explore my limits as well as push them further.

I like intellectual conversations.

My ambition is self-actualisation, to release the potential within.

I'm thoughtful, devoted, industrious, competitive, genuine and trustworthy.

I'm looking to learn and grow, not just to play....

THE END

Other Books by Phil G Include:

*The Absolutely Essential Book of BDSM and S&M Rules
*Things To Do During 3 Hours of Sex; A Step-by-step Guide
*Playtime At The Dom Den; A Step-by-step Guide
*The Absolutely Essential Guide to Great BDSM and S&M Sex
*The Absolutely Essential Dominant/submissive Playtime Experience
*The Absolutely Essential BDSM Sexual Experience
*The Ultimate Collection of S&M and BDSM Rules For Female Submissives and Slaves
*Master and submissive or slave BDSM Contract
*Mistress/slave BDSM Contract
*The Funniest BDSM Personal Ads
*Have Awesome BDSM Sex
*BDSM Master/slave Contract
*Spanking Dictionary
*BDSM Rules
*Bed Arrest, the Punishment for BDSM Enthusiasts

Book #2
Bed Arrest, the Punishment for BDSM Enthusiasts

By Phil G.

Copyright (C) 2013

Trust, care, mutual consent, safe sex practices, and general safety are absolute priorities. No matter what it's suggested that you incorporate at least the following into your playtime and lifestyle:

* Don't tie things around someone's neck, and no breath play, period!
* Create a "Safe word" for the submissive to say when (or if) things get too scary.
* Always be careful and take necessary safety precautions when engaging in BDSM activity. Keep proper medical facilities handy.
* Always insure that a bound person has adequate circulation. If the person tied up has to go to the bathroom or has physical problems, that person must be immediately released from bondage.
* Ask about medical issues before playing and adjust your playing activities according to any medical issues.
* Never leave anyone bound and alone.
* Understand what a gagged person sounds like in sexual ecstasy versus in pain.
* Do not play while under the influence of drugs or alcohol.
Always check that your handcuffs and/or lock keys work before playing. If you have to go to the locksmith to get the handcuffs off, it's going to be embarrassing.
* When removing someone from bondage, allow them to move their own limbs.
* If pregnant or ill, check with your doctor before engaging in BDSM related activity.
* Always play within your own skill base and comfort level.

Bed Arrest, the Punishment for BDSM Enthusiasts

Defining Bed Arrest

Thank you for reading this book, the first book on bed arrest.

This punishment technique can only be used when all parties involved have fully consented to it.

For consistency's sake, this book discusses bed arrest where the punisher is a male master and the person being sentenced to bed arrest is a female submissive or slave. Bed arrest as a punishment can however work just as well in situations when the two parties involved are of the same sex.

I am honored to say that as a master I have incorporated bed arrest into my relationships many times. I have found that it can be a useful tool for changing errant sub/slave behavior.

In this book I'll also make suggestions regarding how (in my opinion) to most optimally carry out the sentence of bed arrest on a sub/slave. Obviously both parties involved can adapt what's in this book to fit their desires, needs and time schedule.

This book also assumes (for all involved) that the sub/slave will accept being put in bed arrest and obey her master's rules associated with it. Obviously if master tells his sub/slave she's just been sentenced to 10 hours house arrest and she points at him and laughs, then master has a problem.

General Definition - Bed arrest is when a master in a BDSM (or related) relationship orders (thus requires) his sub/slave to stay on her bed at all times other than emergencies, and for those additional activities specified. During the time that she is reprimanded to the bed, master may also punish her in other ways such as spanking. He can also play with her, and of course enjoy her sexually.

Bed arrest, as is obvious, is a lot like an adult version of timeout. It doesn't need to be for a longtime; a 30 minute bed arrest session might get the point across just as well. Still all bed arrests sessions are not the same and the sub's restrictions during her incarceration can make all the difference in the world. However beware guys, with her helplessly stuck there, will you be able to resist playing with her all afternoon? (Let's hope she doesn't consider that punishment.)

During bed arrest her freedom can be seriously restricted and she will have time to think about the importance of changing her errant ways.

I gave many 2 day sentences as well as 30 minute sentences. The longest bed arrest sentence I ever given a sub/slave was 4 days. On many occasions I commuted the sentence down because of good behavior, and/or something unexpected came up and/or her sexy begging finally got to me.

Bed arrest in and of itself might not be considered that extreme a punishment. The liberties that the sub/slave loses during bed arrest as well as other punishments she might also experience during that time perhaps can better determine how well she learns her lesson.

1. When to use bed arrest as a punishment. Perhaps your lovely lady has not been reacting well enough to your usual punishments. Perhaps spanking her used to work well as a punishment but now she gets so turned on by it that if anything she'll misbehave to get a good spanking. Finding a new punishment thus has become a necessity.

2. Length of time for putting the sub/slave in bed arrest. Obviously this varies by what extent she needs to be punished and what her and her master's obligations in life are during that time. (Does she have to go to work? Does she have college classes, etc.?)

As she will be allowed out of the bed (and home) for work and other responsibilities, likely that would mean an increase in the length of her sentence as she would be spending less time in bed arrest overall than a sub/slave that could stay around the home all or most of the day.

My experience (and yours may be quite different) is that if the sub/slave has never served a bed arrest, she may have fantasies associated with it.

3. What the sub/slave is allowed to do during bed arrest – How strict and restrictive will her sentence be, at least for the first half or so? Will she need permission to leave the bed for any reason (with the obvious exception of emergencies) including going to the bathroom?

The general rule of thumb is that the less you allow her to do during bed arrest, the more effective the punishment. During the sentence master can progressively give her back more privileges, such as no longer needing permission to go to the bathroom, watch TV, play videogames, watch movies, read books, use the phone, etc. Also was she tied to the bed at all times? Maybe now she can be unbound. (I would strongly suggest that except for emergencies she is never allowed to use the phone during bed arrest.)

My experience is that it's best to start the bed arrest with her having as few privileges as possible and being bound securely to the bed. You then give privileges back as she earns them and/or begs enough for them.

As it's likely you will let her out of the bed to fix meals and do other chores, you'll then need to make sure she's not taking unusually long to do those activities. If so master may want to threaten her with extending her sentence or perhaps another good spanking will take care of that problem.

4. Bondage and blindfolding during her incarceration. Will she be tied up and/or tied to the bed in bondage for a significant amount of the sentence? I would suggest she is and for a substantial amount of time, at least in the first half or more of her incarceration. Blindfolds can help make her feel more isolated and increase the impact of the punishment. Master will probably want to tie her hands in manner so that she **can't** take the blindfold off when she thinks master is not looking, or at least lower the blindfold a bit to look around real quick. Obviously a respectful, well trained sub/slave should not do this but sub/slaves are after all human.

5) Sub/slave needing permission from her master to leave the bed for anything (other than emergencies.) It may seem harsh but my experience is that bed arrest as a punishment works best when to leave the bed for even essential activities, such as going to the bathroom, the sub/slave first needs to have permission from her master. Because of this the master will find that he will need to be in the dwelling and at earshot at all times, just incase, which obviously could be inconvenient for him. With good behavior on her part, this restriction can be lessened.

6) Master will always determine what she does or doesn't wear during the period of bed arrest. *(This is of course is subject to how cold it is, if company shows up and/or if she has to go out of the house for work or other essential activities.)*

During bed arrest, while in private, it's suggested that she not be allowed to wear any clothing.

During the period of her incarceration, also perhaps remove her authority to wear panties while she is out of the house/apartment doing essential public activities such as work and shopping. *(Don't be surprised if she won't go along with this, particularly if it entails doing this at work. If that's the case guys, let it go.)*

7) Pouting, sulking and possibly rebelling by the sub/slave. Master should prepare for his sub/slave to possibly pout, sulk, and as a lengthy sentence progresses, maybe even try to rebel, though hopefully without going too far. Of course the more time master spends with her in bed, playing with her, spanking her, taking her being massaged by her, lying in bed with her, the happier she'll likely be but perhaps the punishment will be less effective, (or perhaps it could have just the opposite effect and be of good benefit).

It's possible that she will rebel to the point that she says she hates you and leaves the house frustrated. It is her right guys and you can't stop her, unfortunately it's likely also a sign of problems in the relationship, and/or a poorly trained sub/slave and/or a sub/slave that simply does not allow herself to be punished with bed arrest, (and/or perhaps other punishments you include during bed arrest.)

Still perhaps she has had a bad experience with bed arrest in the past? That will have to be dealt with in a responsible, respectful manner.

What if she doesn't like bondage and/or blindfolding then either she takes the plunge and lets you do that to her or you don't do those activities.

Perhaps she has obligations that she feels will interfere with the length of her sentence. You would need to let her off for those obligations anyway and perhaps she doesn't understand that.

On the other hand you as master might now find out that she is not a respectful sub/slave, an immature sub/slave and/or too much of a bratty sub/slave and you should find another.

8) Adding more time to her sentence as well as commuting her sentence. The sub/slave should be aware that more time can be added to her sentence. Additionally privileges might not be returned to her as fast during her sentence if she continues to be a bad girl and/or doesn't seem to be learning her lesson.

On the other hand, if she displays a respectful attitude and takes her punishment respectfully then the opposite can occur. Time can be taken off her sentence, and privileges can be returned more quickly during her sentence.

9. How often can we play while she is in bed arrest? Well guys, she's tied up to the bed, naked and blindfolded, good luck keeping your hands off of her! Still the master isn't the one being punished here so his needs and pleasure shouldn't suffer. If he wants his sub/slave to massage him, she should massage him. If he wants fellatio from his sub/slave, by all means get it. If he wants to take his slave, by all means take her. Still it breaks the monotony for her which might not be as conducive to punishment. But it will likely will give her pleasure, make her feel more wanted and loved. Hopefully that won't interfere with her learning her lesson and it might in fact help. Perhaps playing with her later during her incarceration is the better choice, if the master can hold out that long.

Hopefully throughout her sentence she will be on her best behavior in an attempt to get her sentence reduced.

10. What activities can the sub/slave do while she is in bed arrest?

A) Of course her work and parental responsibilities are fully allowed. (If you're living with kids, as you can imagine this punishment could be difficult to perform.)

Still master must watch to make sure she doesn't spend more time than she ordinarily would with her responsibilities. When that's the case her master may wish to add time to her incarceration and/or punish her in other ways.

B) She is required to satisfy her master's sexual desires as always as well as any other activities that can be performed on the bed that she would ordinarily do for her master. This includes massaging her master.

C) Her master perhaps may still also want to punish her in one or more other manners.

11. Privileges that can be taken away from the sub/slave during bed arrest include (depending on circumstances):

*Being able to enjoy video entertainment such as playing video games, watching videos, TV, movies, etc. That can include her favorite programming that would come on during her period of incarceration. (It can be recorded to be watched after her sentence is over.)

*Being able to talk (unless there is an emergency) or she needs permission to do something.

*Being able to use the phone.

*Being able to write things by hand.

*Being able to read for entertainment, such as books.

*Being allowed to have orgasms or otherwise pleasure herself (but dude that's harsh!)

12. Do you close the door on her during her confinement?
No, but it's the master's choice if she's allowed to look at him.

13. How to react to her begging during incarceration. If your sub/slave is adept at begging and if they can be real sexy while doing it, masters may have to ban begging during bed arrest altogether or deal with the horniness that comes with it.

I for one like it when she begs and you can require a certain number of "begs" from her before you'll even consider commuting her sentence.

14. Additional punishments while she is in bed arrest. Perhaps you would like to give her "hourlies". These are spankings given every hour during a set period. She needs to make sure that her master knows it is time for her hourly spanking (or other prescribed hourly punishment) or risk having addition time added to her sentence.

15. Additional general advice to the master. Guys you need to hold strong and be firm. That can be tough. Make sure she takes you seriously throughout this period.

The End

_____

_____

Other Books by Phil G Include:

*The Absolutely Essential Book of BDSM and S&M Rules
*Things To Do During 3 Hours of Sex; A Step-by-step Guide
*Playtime At The Dom Den; A Step-by-step Guide
*The Absolutely Essential Guide to Great BDSM and S&M Sex
*The Absolutely Essential Dominant/submissive Playtime Experience
*The Absolutely Essential BDSM Sexual Experience
*The Ultimate Collection of S&M and BDSM Rules For Female Submissives and Slaves
*Master and submissive or slave BDSM Contract
*Mistress/slave BDSM Contract
*The Funniest BDSM Personal Ads
*Have Awesome BDSM Sex
*BDSM Master/slave Contract
*Spanking Dictionary
*BDSM Rules
*Bed Arrest, the Punishment for BDSM Enthusiasts

This book is sold and/or distributed with the understanding that the publisher and author is not engaged in rendering legal or other professional services, including nutritional and dieting services. **This book and its subject matter are for entertainment purposes only.** Everything in the book should be verified before implementing. In this publication there may be inadvertent inaccuracies including technical inaccuracies, typographical inaccuracies and other possible inaccuracies. **The writer and publisher of this publication expressly disclaim all liability for the use or interpretation by anybody of information contained in this publication.** The author, publisher and distributors of this publication hereby disclaim any and all liability for any loss or damage caused by errors or omissions resulted from negligence, accident, or any other causes. If legal advice or other expert assistance is required, the services of a competent professional person in a consultation capacity should be sought. Products, services and websites' content vary with time. Please verify any published information.

Book #3 – Dramatic Weight Loss Using BDSM

By Phil G.

Copyright (C) 2013

Introduction

BDSM is uniquely qualified to help people lose weight. I'm personally familiar with many women who have successfully lost a surprising amount of weight using this system.

If you are not familiar with BDSM (*Bondage, Discipline, Sadism and/or Masochism,*) please do an Internet search or otherwise learn it better (should that be your wish.) This book has been written primarily for those well acquainted with the lifestyle.

As you know losing weight is an arduous, restrictive, sacrifice-filled experience that isn't particularly fun. To fight this, the dieter needs a lot of motivation. Happily BDSM can be of great service regarding that.

In this book, for simplicity's sake, the dieter is going to be a submissive female and the dieting taskmaster is going to be a dominant male (as well as her Dominant.) Obviously the sexes can be reversed, or instead both parties can be the same sex.

Integral to successful weight loss using BDSM is that the dieter needs to be submissive to the Dominant and relinquish control to him of those aspects of her life that affect her weight loss, such as her dieting. (Case studies are presented later in this book.)

As a Master I have overseen many female submissive/slave's BDSM weight loss programs, and often with very good success. There is no doubt that this kind of BDSM weight loss program can be a first rate weight loss plan. It has proven itself many times.

The biggest problems however are that the dieter (the submissive):

(a) Decides against continuing with the restrictions of the weight loss program (such as the diet)
(b) Rebels against the dominance of her Dominant. (If this occurs, likely all is lost.)

Talk to each other about this in the beginning and again as necessary. Be prepared for it so you can talk about it when (and if) it occurs.

In this weight loss program the dominant will exercise strict control over what she (the submissive) eats and will punish her for infractions as he feels is necessary. She can't rebel against this or the weight loss program likely won't succeed.

She also needs to be honest with herself and to her Dom. She can't go about eating foods (or excess amounts of food) that she isn't allowed to, and/or lie about it, etc. Should she fail regarding this, she should be punished and she needs to accept that.

Unfortunately during the BDSM Weight Loss Program one or more of these problems can manifest themselves:

A) Life throws her a curve ball and she (the dieter) has to get off the weight loss program. In that case let it go and restart it ASAP.

B) Women just don't like to be told they're overweight no matter how true it is, so even discussing it can be a sensitive subject, and that includes while the BDSM Weight Loss Program is going on! *It's very helpful if the woman works past this as it's natural during this time to think that her Dominant has a negative view of her current possibly overweight body.*

I can think of a particular time I put a slave on a BDSM weight loss program and she rebelled after only around 6 days. I'm confident it was not my fault. We ended up ending our online relationship because of this. I was in contact with her a couple of months later and happily she had restarted dieting and had lost a significant amount of weight.

Even though it was me who had finally inspired *and required* her to get on a weight loss program of any sort, she did not in any way associate her weight-loss success with me anymore at that point (and unfairly in my opinion.)

C) The Dominant is not good at this and the submissive needs to break it off due to that. Perhaps he's not a good Dom to start out with or she doesn't respect him as much as both had thought she did. (It helps if the Dom is in decent physical shape and exercises himself but that is comparatively minor.)

The Dominant needs to know how much (and how hard) to push her but if she is sensitive to this type of control then the program is likely doomed to failure.

D) She doesn't want to lose weight bad enough.

E) She rebels against certain specific demands of this strict regimen.

Beware dominants, as previously noted, your relationship with this submissive can readily end because of enforcing the BDSM Weight Loss Program. If she gives up on the program the Dominant can push her to continue but at some point he had best give up or the relationship will almost certainly suffer. I have lost more than one lady because I didn't give up fast enough (though actually it was more because she gave up on the weight loss program too quickly in my opinion.)

What To Do To Implement
The BDSM Weight Loss Program

A) To start out with, the submissive needs to accept that she needs to lose weight. (Hopefully she adamantly wants to lose weight.) The other option is that her Dom/Domme has told her to and she is going to obey him.

B) She might first try the usual methods of losing and keeping weight off, and hopefully that works. If those attempts aren't fruitful enough, or if she wants to try another type of weight loss program from the get-go, then the *BDSM Weight Loss Program* is definitely a way to go.

C) If possible, determine just what the weight loss program's specifics will be. It doesn't need to be complex or extreme.

BDSM weight loss typically is a combination of exercise, good sleep, an acceptable level of stress and diet/calorie restrictions. The more sex she can have during this time, typically the better. Does she have a convenient way to exercise? Does she know where to get low calorie food?

The lack of optimal gut microbes have been tentatively linked to many overweight people are so perhaps a PROBIOTIC should be taken but beware, most, if not all of the live bacteria in a PROBIOTIC supplement is killed by stomach acid so get one that can best survive stomach acid on its way to the colon where it has important work to do. Low calorie yogurt has at least somewhat of a PROBIOTIC EFFECT.

D) Can she afford Nutrisystems, Jenny Craig, Weight Watchers, Medifast or something of that nature? If so you'll likely want to go with that.

E) Does she understand nutrition well enough to know the allowable foods to eat? Most women do. If not her Dom will have to have even stricter control over the food she eats.

F) Tell the sub/slave on what day the program begins. Give her at least one day to party a bit and experience the culinary freedom that she won't have for some time.

G) Maintenance spankings can be a good idea during the weight loss program. This helps the submissive's conscious and/or subconscious mind remember the importance of respecting her commitment to the program and the authority of her Dom who will oversee it and punish her (and reward her) when she fails to keep her end of the bargain.

Definition of a Maintenance Spanking: Spankings administered on a regular basis to keep the spankee on the straight and narrow. (Punishment spankings are administered in addition to these.)

H) Provide encouragement for the submissive and perhaps give her extra time to work out by doing certain chores that take up her time and/or energy.

I) At some point down the road she can start increasing her calorie intake but that should be after significant weight loss or if there are health issues.

J) In most cases it's helpful for weight loss if she speeds up her metabolism in some healthy way.

K) Important, don't forget about rewarding her for her weight loss accomplishments. Be liberal with the rewards. She'll likely really appreciate those and rewards may be the difference in the success or failure of her adherence to the program. I personally would not include higher calorie treats as a reward but it's up to you. The truth is that the sub/slave typically will really look forward to her rewards (though the bigger ones need to be substantial, like a night out or a new special article of clothing, etc.) The sub/slave should feel free to remind her Dom about the rewards from time to time and if the Dom is not rewarding her in a noticeable and significant manner, it's my opinion that he is not keeping up his end of the bargain.

Be generous with minor rewards like watching something she wants to on TV or fixing a nice low calorie dinner for her if the Dom doesn't normally do that. Throw in bigger rewards periodically. Perhaps it is she who should choose, or at least recommend the upcoming reward. (I think it can be better when it is she who chooses at least the major rewards.)

Rule: Rewards cannot be taken away as punishment. She has to be able to take her punishment like a good girl and once she's been punished, it's over. The slate has been wiped clean because she paid fully for her transgression thanks to the punishment. I for one will only supervise a BDSM Weight Loss Program where I can punish her at will. Having a corner to send her to stand in after her well deserved spanking is also a great idea! (If she won't let you spank her then I suspect this weight loss program is not for you two, or it's a long distance relationship.)

Getting her a new sex toy(s) can be a good reward. (As a Dom I require my slave to have a huge amount of sexual pleasure from playing so new sex toys work nicely.)

As a reward, periodically you should take her out to eat where she can have a moderate calorie meal.

L) *Compliments* – We all know how much women love compliments. Doms, don't forget to compliment her for her hard work regarding the weight loss program.

It will also be very helpful if she has a dieting and/or workout support system with family and/or friends. Two or more women starting a weight loss program together is often a great thing, maybe even throw in a bet as to who would be the first to quit.

Perhaps the Dom and sub/slave would like to do this together, both going on at least a diet. A problem is that the Dom can't get punished as readily for transgressions (or can he?) Perhaps he can lower his calorie intake out of respect for what she's going through particularly if they live together.

Her overweight friends and family that don't want to deal with the concept of weight loss can be a problem. They might tell her she looks fine and that she shouldn't feel she needs to work out and/or diet due to their own insecurity and/or laziness. That position however is not good for our situation.

Rules for the Submissive
During the DSM Weight Loss Program

1) The dieter will report specifics (via email or phone) *every* night as to what she ate that day/night and what weight loss activities she engaged in. (It's kind of a diary.) As is obvious, this way her Dom can better keep an eye on her activities.

2) If she wants to eat more than a heaping tablespoon of any higher calorie food, she MUST first get permission from her Dom. (*Her Dom needs to give examples of what "higher calorie food" is.*) For example, if there is an unexpected office party and cake is served, she would need to steal away and call up her Dom and ask permission to have a small slice. (To review, up to a heaping tablespoon in a multi-hour time period never needs permission. More than that *always* needs permission.)

3) Skipping workouts (assuming workouts are part of the program, which ideally they should be) are not allowed unless she has an excellent excuse. (Having a stationary bicycle and/or Stairmaster type of exercise device where she lives can work very well and is convenient. Often thrift stores have these.) **To skip a workout, or not to workout hard enough, she needs permission from her Dom unless there is a health issue**. If she misses a workout for a less than suitable reason, or her workouts are not of an acceptable nature and/or intensity, *she should be punished*!

4) To the Doms reading this, during a lasting weight loss program your resolve will almost certainly be tested by your submissive and you must be prepared to follow through with the threat of punishment, unless she has a good excuse or there are health concerns.

It's very important that she respect you as the administrator of the weight loss program and enforcer of the weight loss program's admittedly arduous restrictions.

It is also a rule that she must accept her punishment.

If you announce a punishment and she balks then chances are either the punishment is unreasonable or she just isn't ready for weight loss the BDSM way.

5) If the dieter has health concerns then the weight loss program is at least suspended. All health concerns must be taken seriously and addressed immediately!

Case Study #1

Lori started the BDSM weight loss program under my guidance. She formerly was my slave (but wasn't at that time.) She still had a strong respect for me as a Dominant though and we played semi-regularly. (As amazing as it sounds, I'm proud to say we actually had an amicable break-up. Yes amicable break-ups really can happen!)

Day #1 – During the previous day she partier with her son. That night she had a sugary soft drink, several slices of regular pizza, salad from the salad bar with a very generous helping of higher calorie salad dressing. Later they had ice cream cones.

The program started the next day with weighing herself after defecating (but before eating.)

Lori could afford Nutrisystem, had preordered and was able to start eating those that day. She had a stationary bicycle in her living room.

We did not live together but were in the same vicinity so we could see each other in person without too much trouble (especially since I lived alone and was self-employed.)

That day she only ate Nutrisystems meals and exercised on the stationary bike for 10 minutes. (She hadn't used the stationary bike in a while.)

We talked on the phone that night and she reported what she ate and told me about her workout. Clearly it was an excellent start for her.

Day #2-4: Nothing eventful. She kept to the plan and reported every night what she did in regard to exer-cycling, walking around the neighborhood and eating. As she was eating Nutrisystems it was easier for her to report her meals. She just needed to say "Nutrisystem meals".

Day #5: She had gone out that night with girlfriends and had 2 Kuala's with crème (the very tasty alcoholic beverage.) This was a problem as she at least needed to call me to ask permission to have the second higher than normal calorie drink, which she didn't. (Frankly having a lower calorie alcoholic beverage would have been better.)

I explained to her how what she did was wrong (which she knew) and had her come over to my place the next day for punishment.

Now is an important time. She might take more diet damaging liberties if her subconscious doesn't realize she can't get away with it. So punishment it would be and frankly it turned us both on anyway☺

I waited alone in my house and she came over while her son was in school. As was standard with us, she was only allowed to wear a skirt or dress when we're together (this dress I picked out for her over the phone last night.) As usual, upon entering she was required to remove her panties and leave them in a dresser by the door. (None of my slaves are allowed to wear panties in my home except for emergencies and when leaving.) She knelt down in front of me and I proceeded to scold her for not abiding by the diet rules. I opened her dress top and played with her breasts while she promised to be good and apologized. I then had her stand up and remove her dress, then kneel down again so I could tie her hands together. She was ordered to lie across my lap so I could give her a good spanking. I used a strap, a slapper and a small paddle and reddened her butt nicely. She made yelps, squirmed and kicked her feet. I then ordered her to stand in the corner, periodically coming over and spanking her while she was there. She once again promised to adhere to the rules. I then ordered her into the bedroom where we had sex and otherwise played for several hours. During our playtime her hands remained tied together.

It was that day that I instigated maintenance spankings every 3 days (if convenient for her, though sometimes it wasn't as we didn't live together and she lived with her son as a single mother.)

Day #6 – Lori's morning weigh in showed she had lost 3 pounds since beginning the diet. She was real happy about it. I thought I saw a difference in her yesterday and had told her that. She called during lunch and wanted to know if she could have the lasagna for lunch at the restaurant but I wouldn't allow it.

That night she emailed me what she ate and drank that day. She also described her workout. She said that she worked out at home with her 7 year old son and they had a good time working out together.

Day #7 – Nothing eventful.

Day #8 – Lori comes over for a maintenance spanking and of course we have sex. Like my punishment spankings her bottom is made red, though not as red as a punishment spanking. I use a variety of spanking implements too. (It's always been my rule that a slave has no more than 60 seconds to be wet from a spanking. No spanking even has the chance of ending until she's wet [with the exception of emergencies of course.])

Lori could take a hard spanking so the red bottom I would make sure to give her before the spanking was over, might be too hard for some other ladies to take. Lori remembered fondly how a paddle broke on her butt at a spanking party.

Day #9 – Lori reports that the dress she initially put on for work was loose, loose enough to make her feel uncomfortable. She had forgotten to weigh herself before eating breakfast so no new weigh-in but we anticipated good news. She sent an email late that night jokingly noting the heaping tablespoon of her son's ice cream she had. She wrote that her workout was 20 minutes on the stationary bicycle and it made her work up a good sweat.

Day #10 – Lori weighs herself after defecating and has lost 6 pounds since beginning the diet. At work already her weight loss was getting noticed and compliments were being handed out. When people ask her how she was doing it she just said

Nutrisystems and exercising, primarily on her stationary bicycle. (It could get her in trouble at work to bring up the BDSM thing.)

Day #11 – This is maintenance spanking day but Lori couldn't get a babysitter so it didn't happen. She was in a bad mood though and my frustration about her not coming over upset her. Fortunately I soothed things over before the conversation ended.

Day #12 – Lori calls that night and wants to eat a small slice of her sister's peach pie which I let her do. She forgot to send me the nightly email report. I told her to come over for punishment ASAP. She apologized and tried to get a babysitter but couldn't find one until two nights later on day #14.

Day #13 – I realized I had not rewarded her yet with anything significant (actually she reminded me over the phone) and I felt bad. The next night she had her babysitter and we went to a Native American casino and I gave her $50 to gamble with, after our meal at the buffet. (As you can imagine I watched her like a hawk as she took food.) We got back to my place and I gave her the maintenance spanking she very much needed, leaving her lovely bare bottom a beautiful shade of red. We had sex of course.

Day #14-15 – Nothing eventful.

Day #16 – Lori weigh-in showed she'd lost a total of 9 pounds and frankly her weight loss for a woman in her 30s was even better than anyone expected. She voiced concern about her dwindling clothing supply (that would fit well.) She began wearing skirts and blouses more which made her feel sexier and seemed to adapt better to her shrinking body. She was being noticed in a positive way at work and got the impression it made her look like someone that can get things done, has drive and has follow-through.

She was a bit frustrated by her somewhat shrinking boobs but the shrinkage was minor. The fact was that she had become a darn good advertisement for Nutrisystems and even her mother planned to start using them. (This book however does not necessarily recommend them over other weight loss nutrition programs.)

Little did anyone other than us know that it was also the *BDSM Weight Loss Program* that was working so well, particularly in providing motivation.

Day #17 – She forgot to email me her daily food and activities. I promise to ad an addition 30 spanks during her next maintenance spanking for that.

Day #18 – With her son gone out of town to his grandmother's for the weekend I was able to spend the night over at her place. I give her her maintenance spanking that evening and have a good time playing with her. I blindfolded her and tied her to the bed in tight bondage and left her there for over an hour. I spanked her again and took her as she laid there helplessly tied up.

After finally releasing her, we showered together and she made us a late dinner of which she also ate instead of nutrisystem food. It was Chop suey filled with vegetables. She had around a cup of rice and a good helping of the Chop suey.

The next morning we got up late, I got stuck with a honey-do list of stuff to do at her place which I spent 6 hours doing, then we played. That night we went through all her cloths to see which no longer "looked good" on her due to the weight loss. (I frankly thought more of her cloths looked fine on her than she did.)

We weeded out about 30% of her cloths and put the cloths that she thought were too big in a separate side of the closet. (Happily her sister had a lot of cloths that would fit Lori's progressively more petite body. Her sister had grown out of those several years ago.)

Well I guess now I'll wrap up my report on Lori. Lori did extremely well on the BDSM weight loss diet. I attribute it to these factors:

1) She really wanted to lose weight; it was an obsession to her.
2) Her body could lose weight faster than many other folks. Perhaps she had a faster metabolism.

3) She had been into BDSM for over 6 years and was very comfortable with her role as a slave.

4) She respected me very much as a Dominant and frankly I again became more of a Master to her. I even collared her on day 23. It was another reward for her doing so well.

5) I did a good job as the Dominant. I backed down in more than one occasion where there could have been trouble if I pushed too much harder. I did a good job with her and frankly I can't say that about all the sub/slaves I administered BDSM Weight Loss with.

6) She also relished all the attention and kudos she got and wasn't hurt that much from the jealousy that more overweight women projected on her.

7) She could afford a specialized nutritional program such as Nutrisystems, Jenny Craig, Weight Watchers, Medifast, etc.

8) She wasn't a food addict and did fine not eating that much even when she was around others that were eating.

Case Study #2

Michele was mostly an online/phone slave of mine. She lived about 260 miles away. I pushed her to start the BDSM weight loss program under my guidance as she was overweight. She wasn't my slave but respected me as a Dominant.

Michelle didn't have Nutrisystems or something of that nature so she would have to concentrate on buying low calorie foods. She did however have a fitness club membership that she had paid for but stopped using.

She drove over to my place for the weekend. She got there Friday night and stayed through Sunday afternoon. Saturday is when the BDSM Weight Loss Program started.

We played throughout the weekend and I made sure she did most of the work screwing. She was out of shape but really worked hard during sex which no doubt burned a lot of calories. Of course I kept her bottom well spanked throughout the weekend. I personally think the sub/slave being well spanked helps the weight loss program but I may be wrong.

We spent a good deal of time setting up her meals. We went online to get ideas and got a huge list of low calorie things for her to make. (Of course there are all the pre-made diet TV dinners to buy in the store.)

Something we tried was having her drink A LOT of water to try and fill her stomach up thus countering hunger pains. That had mixed results.

I had a Stairmaster at my house and made her walk and even run on it twice on Saturday and Sunday. While she was naked on the Stairmaster, I stood behind her with a paddle and paddled her when she didn't walk/run fast enough. As previously noted I made her do as much of the work as possible when we had sex and that included sucking on my cock *many times* each day!

While she was with me she was a very good girl but after she left I could only hope she would obey the rules. She planned on visiting me every other weekend so I could see her progress and punish her in person for not adhering to the rules.

Day #3 – She called to complain about how sore she was from our playtime but also to note what she ate.

Day #4 – Nothing eventful. She sent me the nightly email as to what she ate. She said she was still too sore to go to the gym.

Day #5 – Michelle went to her fitness facility and worked out, mostly working her lower body out. I am sad to report however that Michelle called and admitted to eating two donuts today during a work break. She said she was hungry and just couldn't help herself. Being so far away can make punishment difficult and her next visit was a week and a half away. I feared that she would break down and once again too readily eat forbidden foods. I decided she needed to be punished for that now, as well as when she got here.

One always has to wonder how a particular sub/slave will take to being scolded/punished as she could become defensive and call the whole thing off (if that happens then most likely she was not a good candid for successful BDSM weight loss anyway.) I told her that her punishment for now is that she's not allowed to wear panties until further notice. Obviously this meant she could not wear a dress or skirt in public but she usually didn't anyway. Also I would tack on an extra, good spanking with the paddle when she next came to visit. Before she hung up though I told her she could wear panties for her excursions to the fitness club.

Day #6 – Michelle had weighed herself after defecating (and before eating of course) and had lost 3 pounds since the start of the diet. She emailed me the good news! She also told me how she was at work with no panties on, which excited me. I emailed back congratulating her about the weight loss and told her to report what life is like while not wearing panties. That night she called. She told me of her now panty-less life and gave me the report as to what she ate that day, which was very little, so little that I voiced my concern.

Day #7 – Michelle called that evening and wanted to know if she could have a chicken pasta dish at the restaurant she was at with two of her girlfriends. I told her no. She responded to me with silence and I asked her sternly if "she understood young lady?" and she responded with "Yes Sir" and that was that. She later said that one of her girlfriends gave her a hard time for not "splurging" and getting it. Little did her girlfriend know that she wasn't allowed to do it by her "Dom". (To play it safe, it wasn't something Michelle was telling them about either.)

Unfortunately for Michelle, most of her girlfriends had bad eating habits and didn't really care what they looked like. Only one was attractive to start out with. It ended up being a tough night to hang out with her girlfriends. She went home feeling lonely. She called me up and told me of her frustration. I had to give her a pep talk and we had phone sex. I also had to remind her that she had made a commitment to the weight loss program and me, her Dom and she was required to follow through with the commitment. She agreed and felt better. She asked if she could start wearing panties again and I said yes.

(Interestingly the next day one of her girlfriends called and said that Michelle had inspired her and she also was going to try and lose weight, starting with dieting.)

Day #8 – Michelle had gotten into eating raw vegetables with low calorie salad dressing. She also drank pure fruit juice and went to her fitness club to work out. She however forgot to send me her nightly report of what she ate and did for weight loss. She did however the next morning before she went to work (she worked that Saturday) and so I let it slide.

Day #9 – She called to chat and sounded like she was having a lazy Sunday. I was busy and said she should go work out and call me back when she returned. A few hours later she did but she sounded irritable. I finally asked her if she was feeling okay and/or if she was mad about something. She finally said that it frustrated her that I didn't want her the way she was and it seemed that I would only want her if she was the slender "Barbie doll type".

Well this took me by surprise but this is a common way for the lady in the BDSM weight loss program to act and feel, at least periodically.

The truth was I wanted her to look better and be more sexy, the way that more slender women often are. Was I to be blamed for that? The truth was that as a guy I wanted her to be truly height weight proportionate, which she wasn't yet. For some reason I was however not allowed to think that way or was not allowed to take those thoughts seriously. (I certainly was not allowed to voice this desire.)

I had been here before and had told the truth to women which was that I would find her more attractive if she was a more optimal weight, but that offended the women and the relationship always had ended, at least for purposes of the BDSM Weight Loss Program.

Guys now is the time for you to perhaps swallow your pride and perhaps tell a little "white lie", that being that you thought she was just as attractive and desirable now as she would be when she became height weight proportionate, or better yet slender. She wants to hear that and her shot at serious weight loss from the BDSM diet could be lost if you don't.

The truth is I have a good deal of experience administering the BDSM Weight Loss Program and this obstacle comes up *a lot*.

I told Michelle that she just wasn't all she could be and I took this weight loss program very seriously and she should also. It was being done for *her*. I also told her what a fine person she was and that I was sexually attracted to her.

I don't know if she believed me but the phone conversation ended in a somewhat tense manner. I never heard from her that night with her nightly report though and neither of us communicated with each other for a number of days.

Her BDSM Weight Loss Program was over as was our romantic relationship.

Epilogue

The premise of the weight loss program is pretty straight forward. How long she stays with the program is another story.

Both parties should be prepared for the additional competition for her affections that can come into play as she loses weight.

Best of luck to all.

The End

Other Books by Phil G Include:

The Absolutely Essential Book of BDSM and S&M Rules
Things To Do During 3 Hours of Sex; A Step-by-step Guide
Playtime At The Dom Den; A Step-by-step Guide
The Absolutely Essential Guide to Great BDSM and S&M Sex
The Absolutely Essential Dominant/submissive Playtime Experience
The Absolutely Essential BDSM Sexual Experience
The Ultimate Collection of S&M and BDSM Rules For Female Submissives and Slaves
Master and submissive or slave BDSM Contract
Mistress/slave BDSM Contract
The World's Most Entertaining Kinky Personal Ads
The Funniest BDSM Personal Ads
Have Awesome BDSM Sex
BDSM Master/slave Contract
Spanking Dictionary
BDSM Rules
Bed Arrest, the Punishment for BDSM Enthusiasts

Book #4
Absolutely Essential Tips For Buying & Selling On eBay

Absolutely Essential Tips For Buying & Selling On eBay

Important Tips for Buying on eBay

1) Last Minute Bidding Frenzies - Perhaps you've noticed that often there's a bidding frenzy in the last one minute of bidding. New bidders may suddenly start bidding in the hope that the previous bidders will not be watching or can't increase their bid in time. Often however it's because of *Sniping*.

Sniping websites automatically bid on your behalf, often in the last 10ish seconds. Simply sign up, enter an eBay item number and the maximum price you're willing to pay. Hidbid.com and goofbid.com offer sniping services that place bids for you.

Typically you'll need to give sniping sites your eBay password for them to work (ugh!!) Obviously that is a serious security concern.

There's little protection from eBay if things go wrong when sniping, since you willingly gave your password to a third party. If you do sign up for such a service, never use the same password for eBay as you use for other accounts like banks accounts or email addresses.

2) Second-chance Auction Scams, Beware of Them - Unscrupulous people sometimes watch bidders in high-dollar auctions and try to take unsuspecting buyer's money after an auction ends.

The scheme, known as a *Second-chance Auction Scam*, is just one of many types of Internet auction frauds reported to the *Internet Crime Complaint Center,* or *IC3*.

Second-chance scammers wait until auctions end and then offer bidders that lost, a phony second chance to purchase the item -- usually through a wire transfer service. This happens more often than people realize, beware!

3) Misspelling Search Tool - Typojoe.com, goofbid.com, bargainchecker.com, fatfingers.co.uk and baycrazy.com - There are many items listed on eBay every day that have misspelled words in the title. It's unfortunate for the seller but chances are good those listings will not come up well in eBay's search engine (because misspelling causes keyword problems) and thus not bring the seller top dollar. Their loss can be your gain!

4) Bidding Tip - Often sellers start auctions at .99 cents, (or at least under a dollar) hoping a bidding war will erupt. Many items go unspotted, staying at this super-low price (99 cents). *LastminuteAuction.com* hunts for eBay auctions due to finish within an hour but where the price still is very low.

With these items in particular, double-check delivery charges, as some sellers hope to recoup costs by charging a little extra (though eBay's now set maximum delivery charges for many categories).

5) Don't Forget About Facebook - *Facebook Marketplace* is a force to be reckoned with. Also sellers often are open to haggling. Just log on to your account at Facebook and search for "Marketplace". It's also worth checking to see if there's any local Facebook selling groups in your area.

6) Nigerian Type Scam for Paying. These unscrupulous people want to pay with a money order that they claim to already have handy. Often it's for more than the purchase amount. He writes to ask if the seller would be "honest enough" (or something of that nature) to send him the extra cash along with the item. (However he might just try to only buy the item with it and not ask for extra cash.) Unfortunately the money order can look okay but is counterfeit. They particularly like the *Buy It Now* feature.

7) Set Long-term Alerts For Rare Items - If you want something very specific or hard to find, set a 'favorite search' and eBay will email each time a seller lists your desired item.

Simply type a product in eBay's search bar, such as "silver dollar", and click 'save search'. Be as specific as possible for the most accurate results. When (and if) someone lists one, you're alerted with an email.

8) Don't Assume eBay's the Cheapest Place To Get Your Item - Many people assume that if it's on eBay, it's automatically the least expensive place to get it, but that often isn't the case. Perhaps you'd also like to use *shopbots* (shopping robots) that check numerous Internet retailers to find the best price. Type into a search engine "shopping comparison sites".

The same rule applies when buying used merchandise. Check used marketplaces on Amazon.com and Play.com - you may even get it for free on Freecycle or Freegle.

9) Check the eBay Going Rate For an Item - There's a quick way to check an eBay product's average price. Enter the item into the search box and click "completed listings". What will come up is a list of prices that similar auctions have already settled on. After that, sort it by "Price: lowest first". If the price is red, it means no one bought it. Green means it sold. Figure out the average price.

10) eBay has banned the selling of intangible items, and that includes curses! - Among the items that were prohibited as of August 30, 2012, are "advice; spells; curses; hexing; conjuring; magic; prayers; blessing services; magic potions; healing sessions; work from home businesses and information; wholesale lists, and drop shop lists."

11) Haggling on eBay Can Pay Off - There's nothing wrong with asking for a discount, even if the listing doesn't have the "make offer" indication. Haggling works best on *Buy It Now* listings, or auctions with a high start price and no bids. Also you'll likely do better if you haggle as the auction is coming closer to closing as the seller could start feeling more desperate.

To contact the seller, click on the seller's nickname then "ask seller a question". If you're polite, you'll likely get further. Blunt requests such as "dude, how about $15?" likely won't work out as well. Remember the seller is likely going to lose money doing this so no point in being annoying.

Once you've arranged a deal, try to keep the transaction within eBay. Ask the seller to add (or change) a Buy It Now price. That way you don't lose the usual eBay buyer protection privileges.

12) Other Things to Do To Exploit Sellers' Screw-ups - Some sellers make basic mistakes, leavings goods going for bargain money.

As well as spelling boo-boos, another error is to leave out key details such as shoe size, dress brand, saying a console's an a Wii when the photo shows a Xbox. At this point, many buyers give it up as "too much hassle".

So contact the seller to fill in gaps, but don't ask the question via the item's listing page, (because that way, when the seller replies, eBay lets them add their reply to the main listing, so it's no longer your secret.)

Instead, ask the question via the seller's profile (make it clear which item you're talking about). They might not bother with the extra hassle of adding it to the listing, so you'll be the only one in the know.

Also the seller might not realize how pricy an item he/she actually has.

13) Tool to Track Down Crazy End Times - Listings that finish at anti-social times often get fewer bids, thus sell for less. To locate auctions that finish when fewer people are around to bid on them, use BayCrazy's *Crazy End Time* search. (A lot more on the best times to end your auction in the next section of the book *"Selling on eBay"*.)

Check out their auto-bidding tools if you don't want to spend all that time in front of the computer bidding at odd times. Other

BayCrazy.com tools include "unwanted gift" and "ending now" searches.
www.baycrazy.com/search.php?page=nightowl (Baycrazy offers other eBay related opportunities also.)

14) Search Descriptions as Well as Titles - eBay automatically searches seller's titles for results that include your specified keywords. If you're not getting the results you want, try also searching the item's *description* too. (To do this go to Advanced Search.)

For example, imagine you were searching for a REI Jacket. Unfortunately the seller may be selling one but only put "Ski Jacket" in the title however he mentioned "REI" in the description. Include description in your search and then it should then come up.

15) Search Using eBay Boolean Logic - If a seller could describe an item different ways, you can make eBay search for several different ways of describing it at once. Just place "(("at the beginning and enter different phrases individually enclosed by quotation marks, then followed by commas.

So for example, type... (("fishing tackle", "hook", "reel" ...and it will simultaneously bring up listings that contain the words "fishing tackle", "hook" and/or "reel".

16) Add A Few Extra Cents to Your Bid - When bidding, you enter a "maximum bid", and eBay makes automatic bids on your behalf up to your maximum bid.

Don't enter a round number. For example, if a coat is currently selling for $20, and the most you are willing to pay for it is $25, enter a maximum bid of $25.24. If someone tries to outbid you by entering the round number of $25, they will receive an outbid notice. eBay will go your bid, even though it's just 24 cents more.

17) Be Somewhat Skeptical of Feedback - eBay sellers have a feedback rating that acts as a useful guide to previous seller's opinion's of them. As a guideline, look for a seller with more than 98% positive feedback and a high feedback score of at least 30. Also ensure you read their feedback from their *selling*, not just their *buying*. (To see their feedback, click on their username).

18) Seller with Zero Feedback Could be Cause For Concern - Think twice before purchasing expensive items from a seller with zero feedback.

Remember feedback's useful but not infallible. One thing to watch for is traders selling a number of cheap things for $1ish each to build their feedback, and suddenly listing items costing hundreds each.

19) Check to Make Sure You're Bidding on the Actual Item - Sometimes you assume you're bidding for an item on eBay (or any auction site,) when all that's actually being sold is a link to another site selling it. People are not suppose to be able to sell these on eBay but they can fall through the cracks.

Always read the whole description in detail before bidding. Often the catch is hidden in the text at the end – an attempt to protect the seller from any recourse.

20) Scam - Beware of it - It's a red flag if a seller writes "Before bidding, contact me" then asks for a money transfer. Thieves who hijack actual eBay accounts might use this tactic.

21) Scam - Beware of it - Always be worried if you're asked to pay by an instant money transfer service such as Western Union or MoneyGram. Instant money transfer payments cannot be traced and are highly popular with thieves.

22) Sneakily Find Underpriced Buy It Nows - Feel free to hunt for Buy It Now bargains also. Perhaps the seller under-values their item making their price a good deal.

These steals are snapped up quickly. Go to "Advanced Search", select a category you're interested in, filter it to show *Buy It Now* items and sort the results.

23) Always Complain within 45 Days - Under eBay's buyer protection program, 45 days is the most number of days you have to open a case if you're unhappy with your purchase. (There are some exceptions such as tickets for events that are months away.) Read more on eBay's protection policy.
http://pages.ebay.com/help/policies/buyer-protection.html#conditions1

Under eBay's own Buyer Protection rules, buyers are eligible for a refund if the item's "not as described", meaning it didn't match the seller's description. http://pages.ebay.com/coverage/index.html

24) Pay by PayPal - Avoid sending checks and never use money orders. It's much harder for scammers to disappear with your cash when you use eBay's online payment system, PayPal.

Paying this way costs the same as paying by check, but means you're covered by eBay's Buyer Protection program. If an item is faulty, counterfeit or non-existent, you are far more likely to get a refund.

25) Outbid? Don't Give Up On It Yet - Missed out on a desired item by pennies? Don't give up hope. As every seller knows, sales sometimes don't materialize when buyers change their minds or can't come up with the dough. Because of that feel free to send a friendly message such as: "Hi, I've been looking for this poster for years and just saw your finished auction. Please let me know if the sale doesn't come through."

They may send a *Second-chance Offer*, which are sent out by sellers to unsuccessful bidders if the winner fails to pay up. Ask them to relist at an agreed *Buy It Now* price.

26) Know Your Consumer Rights - When buying from a person who makes or sells goods for resale on eBay you often have the same rights as when buying in person from a shop that does the same. This means your goods must be of satisfactory quality and as described.

With private sellers it's buyer beware. Buyers' only rights under law are that the product is fairly described and the owner has the right to sell it.

Under eBay's own Buyer Protection rules, buyers are eligible for a refund if the item is "not as described", meaning it doesn't match the seller's description.

27) Beware of All The Fakes - While eBay has a 'flag and remove' policy to help identify fakes, still plenty fall through the cracks.

If you're buying big-name brands, do your research first. Carefully check sellers' feedback and post on the forum's eBay board to get others' opinions. Be especially wary of overseas sellers or branded items that seem especially cheap.

The more *unprofessional* the photos, likely the better. Thieves often take professional photos from the brands' sites. Legitimate sellers typically take photos of items at home that might not come out as well.

28) Think Twice Before You Give A Seller Negative Feedback - Of course, negative feedback is often justified but have a heart, don't leave negative or even *neutral* feedback without first trying to work the issue out with the seller. Most sellers are good folks who will try to help particularly, as it can mean a lot to their business to stay in your good graces.

Remember eBay users can view the feedback you've left for others, and if you leave a significant amount of negative feedback, they may well decide you're too high of a risk to sell to.

29) Add An Item You're Interested in to eBay's "Watch List" - Want to keep track of an item without bidding on it? eBay lets you add items to a "Watch List", so you can relax knowing you'll get an email reminder within 36 hours of the auction ending. To watch an item, just click the "*add to watch list*" link in the upper part of the item's eBay webpage.

30) Don't Do Private Purchasing - Sellers may suggest you do a deal outside eBay for a cheaper price. If you do you'll likely have less protection if things go bad. You won't be able to leave negative feedback and you won't be protected by eBay's Buyer Protection Plan.

31) Think Safety When Picking Up An Item In Person - The usual precautions apply. If you get to their door and the seller's holding a butcher knife, now's the time to run.

32) Think International - There's bargains to be had on overseas eBay sites. To include foreign auctions in search results, click "worldwide" for location.

Still can't find what you want? Another option is buying directly from *international* eBay sites. The main ones are USA, Canada, Australia, Germany, France and Spain - there's a full list at the bottom of eBay's homepage. Make sure that the item reads *"Shipping to: worldwide"* before bidding as some international sellers only do business with their country's buyers.

Always factor in postage and if applicable, custom fees. Remember that return postage fees could be hefty.

Also what kind of credit card protections will there be? You're often still protected by eBay and PayPal's buyer protections (if you use PayPal), but it's worth investigating. Type in "buyer protection" in PayPal.

33) Don't Forget The Online Classified Ads - Again, let's not assume that because it's on eBay, that's where you'll get the best price for an item. Unfortunately that's often just not the case. Type "top classified ad sites" or something of that nature, into search engines. There's also *Freecycle* and *Freegle*. (Those two sites offer free stuff. freecycle.org and ilovefreegle.org.)

Remember, anyone can post on these classified ad sites. If someone asks you to pay by MoneyGram or Western Union, as always be concerned. It's a bad way to pay.

34) Check Other Auction Sites Also - There are other auction sites that can be found through search engines. If you're searching for something specific, it's also worth adding it to your search. *Auctionlotwatch*.com is a useful shopbot for online auctions. Search for an item and it trawls the big auction sites for you.

35) Check Cashback and Voucher Websites - Check cashback websites to see if there's money back available on your eBay purchase. Type into search engines: "cashback and voucher sites".

Cashback sites give you a cut of their proceeds by setting you up with product and/or service providers.

36) eBay has trained teachers that could be in your area. Also see eBay University. Check out:
http://pages.ebay.com/sellerinformation/howtosell/university.html

Important Tips for Selling on eBay

1) Join eBay Forums - Ask questions about anything, selling, buying etc. Great information is posted already and could be of use. Work together as a team. Find eBay and other auction forums by looking those up in search engines. Ebay has forums also. http://forums.ebay.com/category/Ebay-Discussion-Boards/2001

2) eBay Research Tool 1 - To help in your research about selling items, you can go Type into a search engine "best selling eBay items." EBay provides that information.

3) eBay Research Tool 2 - You can use Ebuyers (www.ebuyersedge.com) to just search eBay for items as well as set up a saved eBay search (or a number of them). You'll get alerted with an e-mail when a matching item is listed.

4) Sell Refurbished Products - Refurbished products fall somewhere in between new and used products. Refurbished products are not new, but often they aren't significantly used either. Sometimes a customer buys the product and for whatever reason, returns it for a refund. The item is then returned to the manufacturer, given an inspection, repaired as necessary and sold as refurbished.

There are various ways an item can become refurbished.

1. The packaging of an item can be damaged during shipping. In that case the item is sent back to the seller/manufacturer. Refurbished items usually come with manufacturer's warranties. Although sometimes the warranties that come with refurbished items are for a shorter period of time, the products are usually in very good condition.

2. Items that have a slight defect or flaw, like a scratch or mechanical flaw, might be returned to the manufacturer. The manufacturer repairs the items, repackages them and marks them refurbished.

3. Demonstration units are also considered refurbished, but generally that's when they're returned to the manufacturer, inspected and repackaged.

4. Brand new overstock items can also be marked refurbished.

5. Sometimes it's a situation where only the packaging of an item is opened. It's re-packaged or even just closed up and marked as refurbished.

Refurbished Products Advantages:

a. Refurbished products are significantly cheaper than new products. They also come with warranties, boxes and everything else new products come with.

b. Selling refurbished products is more profitable, even though refurbished products cost significantly less than new products. On eBay (and at other places) refurbished products can sell for the same price as new ones. (Many people buy refurbished products thinking they're buying new ones.)

c. Refurbished products are sometimes new! When you buy a lot of refurbished products they might actually be overstock items or factory overruns. In that case you would be buying new products at a fraction of the price.

Refurbished Products Disadvantages:

a. Refurbished is not new, even though refurbished products can be exactly the same as new ones, people simply prefer new items.

b. Refurbished products are sometimes the previous year's models. If you're selling electronics or computers it could bring the selling prices down.

5) Finding Products To Sell - Unfortunately finding products to sell can be the toughest part of starting your eBay business. Many people end up opting against starting an eBay business because they can't find a good supplier.

a) YELLOWPAGES.COM - www.yellowpages.com. Try this first. Yellowpages.com can find specialized suppliers in your area. Type in "wholesale" into the search box and you will be given a bunch of subdirectories to further explore. Make sure the search is based on a location near you. Next type "wholesale directory" or "wholesale directories" into search engines.

When searching also try inputting keywords such as overstock, salvage, surplus, liquidation, auction, refurbished, refurb, supplier, closeout, wholesale, etc.

b) BUY FROM AN ACTUAL EBAY SELLER. Buy multiple items and get a discount. That discount could be your margin of profit.

c) BUY WHOLESALE LOTS FROM EBAY AND RESALE THEM - Go to eBay and search for "wholesale lot". If you buy a big lot, you could find you profit best by individually selling the items in the big lot.

d) PERHAPS SELL DIGITAL COUPONS. You should be able to get them for free. As of this writing, people are posting that coupons sell well on eBay. If you're selling coupons, you need to mention that your auction is for the time you spend finding, assembling (sorting) and sending the coupons to the buyer rather than selling the coupons themselves. It's illegal to sell coupons and that's why auctions say the payment is for the time to gather and sort them. Still it can take time to find good coupons and first folks need to know where to look.

e) BUY FROM LIQUIDATION COMPANIES - A liquidator is someone that buys overruns from big retailers (Sears, K-mart, Wal-Mart etc.) at a fraction of the wholesale price. Sometimes big stores can't sell everything they have. The stuff they couldn't sell needs to be gotten rid of as soon as possible to make room for new products. This is where liquidation companies come in. They buy the overruns products, often at a fraction of the wholesale price. When a liquidation company buys a couple of truckloads full of overruns, the next thing it must do is sell these overruns ASAP to make room for more overruns. Since the liquidator must get rid of the products as soon as possible, the products are sold at cheap prices and often in bulk. Perhaps there are liquidator stores in your town what would make you a deal and you wouldn't necessarily have to buy in bulk.

f) EBOOK SALES - With ebooks, you can sell a digital product that can simply be emailed to your customer. No packing and shipping involved! Selling ebooks on eBay is easy. In fact there are systems you can implement to essentially automate the entire process. You could do a *Buy It Now* auction, or just start the bidding at a reasonable price. When the auction ends and the buyer pays you, all you need to do is email the eBook to them. Again, that's the great thing about downloadable information products: no packaging or shipping is necessary. Perhaps you'd like to offer an entire collection of eBooks to sell on eBay. You'll need eBooks that you own or have given you resale rights.

g) You can sell peoples' houses, cars, boats, or even jewelry collections. Just look in the for sale listings of your local newspaper and look at all of the great stuff for sale that would sell on eBay. Call up the owners of the items advertised in the newspaper and offer to sell the stuff for them. Looking for stuff in newspapers is great because the people that are using a newspaper to sell something probably know little about eBay and are desperate to get rid of the stuff they're advertising. These people are also the ones that are willing to lower the price and haggle, and that is great because the lower the price they are willing to let the item go for, the more profit you can make by selling their stuff.

h) RUNNING ADS TO FIND MERCHANDISE - You can run ads in print media and/or post what you're looking for in Internet forums with something like "I will buy your stuff". As previously noted, if you are going to use this method you will need to pick a used product that keeps its value well. If you're going to use this method you should buy things like jewelry and watches, antiques and other things that appreciate with age.

A previous seller's success story was selling old collectable Apple computers. This is a type of item that some people have laying around in the basement or attic, and will likely never use again. They're more than happy to unload it and get a little money for it at the same time. But on eBay it was a whole new ballgame. There are thousands of people who collect old collectable computers.

6) Sell To Resellers - Anyone looking to buy products and resell them to make a profit is a very good customer that will come back and buy from you again and again. Plenty of people buy stuff on eBay then resell it on eBay! There are also those who buy products on eBay to resell them on their other ecommerce websites or actual stores they may own. A lot of PowerSellers (special higher volume eBay sellers with a closer relationship to eBay) started by buying stuff off of eBay and simply putting it back up for auction.

7) Order Samples If Possible - This is a particularly good tip if you don't have a chance to inspect and see the products you are ordering in person. Many people starting out on eBay make the mistake of placing a big order before actually seeing what they're ordering. By ordering samples you'll be able to test not only the quality of the products you're ordering but the service, communication and legitimacy of the company you're ordering from. If you're thinking of selling designer clothing on eBay, be extra careful when ordering your supplies from the Internet. There is a lot of fake (counterfeit) clothing being sold on the Internet. Remember the pictures on the supplier's website may look real, but that doesn't mean they will be sending you what's in the picture.

If you find a great deal but the "supplier" won't allow any sample orders and wants you to pay through an untraceable method, be wary.

8) Second-chance Offers - If the buyer of your item falls through, you can send the other bidders a *Second-chance Offer* to see if they're still interested in buying it.

9) The Listing's Title - The title of your listing should be clear, relevant to what you are selling and attention grabbing. Always include the correct spelling of the item in the title. Don't try to make the title "cool" by deliberately misspelling words, unless perhaps if the slang name for it is popular. If you misspell the title, your listing won't show up in search results because presumably most people aren't searching for the slang name (or misspelled version) of the product.

The title has to be short (eBay rules), so make sure you include the name of the item and abbreviated descriptions, and try not to waste any space on words that are not needed. *By the same token, always use the entire allotted space to write your title. In general, the longer the title, the better, as long as all your keywords are relevant.*

10) Keywords & Relevancy - Make sure the brand name of what you're selling is in the title! If you're selling a Champion Portable Generator, your listing title should include the make and model number, in this case "New Champion 42431 Portable Generator, 1500 Watt". Your listing title should be a short, abbreviated description of the item you are selling.

The name of the product in the title has to do with the search results (keywords). If people want to buy your portable generator they may search "portable generator, generator, Champion, Champion portable generator," etc. You want to make your listing show up in as many search results as possible.

In review, a wild but catchy title will definitely grab the attention of most people who see it, but won't come up in many people's search results, unless also in the title listing is the name of the product that people would type in when looking for it. (Even that's not guaranteed to work.)

11) If a potential customer wants other people's opinions on a product you sell, you might want to send them to the Amazon.com's webpage for the site as Amazon posts feedback from buyers of that same product. Make sure that Amazon is not selling it for less than you are or that idea could backfire!

12) Mention Flaws: If there is a flaw in the item you are selling, make sure you mention it (though try to call it something else like "scratch" or "mark" if that's what it is.) If your product has a flaw and you don't mention it in your listing, you could get negative feedback and a request for a refund from the person who buys the "flawed" item.

If possible, make the flaw sound positive. You could say "this product has a small dent that has no effects on its operation, but because of this you save big bucks!"

Mentioning a flaw also can make you look like an honest person. You can even have the flaw mentioned in your bullet points - Small scratch on the top (saves you money!!)

13) Host Your Own Pictures - You can host your own pictures on another website or your eBay Store and thus show many, many more photos free of charge.

14) Payment Options: - You should offer the customer several different choices of payment. Most of your customers will pay you through PayPal, (PayPal is owned by eBay,) so make sure you get a PayPal account (www.PayPal.com). Of course, not everyone who buys items on eBay prefers PayPal, some may prefer Western union's Bidpay or another payment system. Another one you should sign up for is StormPay as it can be used by people in some countries where PayPal is not used or as popular. For your free StormPay account go to: stormpay.com.

Wire Transfers - Unscrupulous overseas buyers prefer these as they're not as traceable. It's preferable not to take them.

15) *Offering SquareTrade Warranties* - If applicable to what you're selling, another good way to build trust is to sign up for SquareTrade warranties at www.squaretrade.com. www.squaretrade.com/seller-faq

16) *About Me Page* - The About Me page is often overlooked by many eBay sellers (and buyers.) While having the free About Me page likely will not dramatically increase your sales, it can help if you have good things to say about yourself and a nice picture. Note, many sellers only include links to their listings and maybe not enough information about themselves in the About Me page.

17) *People Bidding with 0 Feedback ratings* - Having a good to great feedback rating is so important as you know. Many sellers refuse letting members with 0 feedback bid on their auctions. Getting a negative feedback from somebody that unpredictable is simply a risk we don't want to take. In many cases, we simply don't trust them.

18) *Best Time To End Your Auction* - The best time for an auction to close (end) is in the evenings and on weekends as that's when most people are on the Internet for that type of activity! You want to make sure that when your auction is closing (ending), everyone that's interested in it is available to bid on it. The mornings are the times that the eBay website gets the least visitors (as people are more often sleeping or working.)

If you live in the Eastern Time Zone, list your auction between 9pm-11pm, Central Time Zone list between 8-10pm, Mountain Time Zone between 7-9pm, and for the Pacific Time Zone list between 6-8pm. This will give you the biggest exposure at the end of your auction. The debate is out as to what day your auction should end on. Some sellers report that Tuesday, Wednesday and Thursday are best. Other sellers report that Saturday and Sunday are best.

There are a few exceptions though. For example, some business products sell best during weekdays and during work hours. Obviously this is because people are usually ordering those types of products at work, for work. Studies have shown that a listing that ends at peak hours can attract up to 25% more bids than one that ends in non-peak hours. Listing your auctions at optimal times is one of the easiest ways to attract more bids.

To end the auction in the evenings, you'll need to put the item for sale in the evening (*or use listing software [see next page] to do it for you*) as eBay considers each day to have a length of 24 hours.

Note, it's eBay's practice that when someone's auction is ending, that listing shows up higher on keyword search results (which is a good thing!)

19) Terms of Service Webpage (Yours) - That's something even a lot of experienced sellers don't seem to include, though it likely won't be necessary if all the information is already in your FAQ webpage. For instance, what's the return policy? What are the shipping options, and what will they cost? What are the accepted methods of payment? How soon is payment to be sent? What is the warranty?

20) Listing Software (For Your Items) - Listing software organizes your eBay listings making the listing part of your business simpler and more efficient. There are many different kinds of listing software. You can do an Internet search for them.

Turbo Lister is free software from eBay. Turbo Lister allows you to upload thousands of listings at a time. It saves listings, schedules your listings and uploads them to eBay automatically. Using it you can edit multiple listings at the same time, preview what your listings will look like before uploading them and more. More eBay software is offered at:
http://pages.ebay.com/help/sell/advanced_selling_tools.html

21) Drop Shipping What You Sell - With drop shipping all you have to do is list items up for auction and when they sell, you contact your supplier, who ships the products from their factory, straight to your customers. In theory drop shipping is a good way to go, but it could offer problems. What happens when you sell items and your supplier sends them to the wrong addresses? What happens when you sell items and your supplier is out of stock? In those cases your reputation suffers. If you are going to use drop shipping; make sure there is good communication between you and your supplier (drop shipper.) Also make sure you have some products in stock in case the supplier runs out by the time your auctions have closed.

22) eBay Stores - eBay stores can be great if you have a number of items to sell. First you'll need to reach the minimum number of feedbacks required (10) to open one. Most PowerSellers have eBay stores. Store sellers can see an increase in profit of up to 25% in the first three months of opening the store (according to eBay). Having your own eBay store can save you a substantial amount of money in listing fees and let you sell items in a fixed price format as well as selling via auctions. Also you can list items for a much longer time and store them in your inventory list for 30, 60, 90, 120 days and even "Good till Cancelled". You'll can feature links to other auctions in all your listings by utilizing a cross promotion tool. There are also bonuses like your own search engine and monthly reports from eBay featuring statistics and dada about your sales in the past month.

An eBay store also gives you a location. It gives you a base of operation, a place where people can easily find you, and a place where repeat customers can come back to. Your customers will be able to bookmark and return to your store, and it may also be indexed in the major search engines. So if you're selling silver dollars, and someone does a BING search for silver dollars, your eBay store may appear in the results along with the usual online retail websites! Obviously this can increase your traffic greatly, and likewise boost your sales.

23) Your eBay Store Identity - Ideally your eBay store should look different from your competition. You can use the design templates eBay offer you, but perhaps it's best to use original graphics. Fortunately eBay Stores are customizable. Ideally, to establish your name, your eBay store should appear like your listings as much as possible. Same colors, design and look.

24) Get a Domain Name - You need to get a simple and memorable domain name. A domain name makes it simple for people to find you. The standard web address eBay will give to your store will look like this: *stores.ebay.com/yourname*, this is not a very memorable web address and it's too long to be easy to type into a web browser. It would be best if you had a web address like *mystore.com*.

The End

Other Books by Phil G Include:

*The Absolutely Essential Book of BDSM and S&M Rules
*Things To Do During 3 Hours of Sex; A Step-by-step Guide
*Playtime At The Dom Den; A Step-by-step Guide
*The Absolutely Essential Guide to Great BDSM and S&M Sex
*The Absolutely Essential Dominant/submissive Playtime Experience
*The Absolutely Essential BDSM Sexual Experience
*The Ultimate Collection of S&M and BDSM Rules For Female Submissives and Slaves
*Master and submissive or slave BDSM Contract
*Mistress/slave BDSM Contract
*The Funniest BDSM Personal Ads
*Have Awesome BDSM Sex
*BDSM Master/slave Contract
*Spanking Dictionary
*BDSM Rules
*Bed Arrest, the Punishment for BDSM Enthusiasts

Book #5
The Absolutely Essential Guide to Erotic Breast Massage

Michelle Talia

Copyright (C) 2013

The Absolutely Essential Guide to Erotic Breast Massage

The specialized breast massage discussed in this book can give a woman a surprising amount of pleasure. If her lover is unavailable to pleasure her this way women can easily give themselves *Extreme Pleasure Breast Massage*, and it's something women can do to themselves for the rest of their lives.

There are a many positions a woman's body can be in to receive this specialized and very sexually arousing breast massage. For this example though, let's have her sitting up and at least topless. Do note however that as she gets more and more aroused, she'd probably prefer to be naked so one or both of you can access her pubic area with fingers or toys while she's experiencing Extreme Pleasure Breast Massage.

For this position the massager sits behind her with his/her chest up against her back. If it's okay with who is getting the massage, I suggest the massager be naked as many women will lose control at some point when getting Extreme Pleasure Breast Massage and be anxiously reaching behind their lower backs to play with the massager's privates. If a woman has never experienced this type of erotic massage before, she in particular may react with callous abandon.

Before placing yourselves in any of the massage positions, you'll need to have readily available a good supply of quality lotion, massage oil or hair conditioner (yes the stuff you might put on your hair. Thicker hair conditioner is often better and the cheaper brands might work just as well.)

If using lotion, try to use some brand of non-desensitizing lotion. (Most lotion's ingredients include desensitizers to dull the pain of dry skin and other irritations. These desensitizers can at least partially desensitize breasts, thus cutting down on the breast's capacity to provide pleasure.) Baby lotions at dollar stores may be good ones to try but lotions tend to vary by brand. Optimally you want the massaging medium to stay slippery as long as possible and, not cause any irritation of course. Cold lotion/oil/conditioner on breasts can provide an unwelcome jolt so if warming is necessary, warm the lotion/oil/conditioner up ahead of time using the microwave oven, or by setting it in hot water. Make sure the top is loosened somewhat incase it warms up too much and creates steam. (You can also rub together blobs of it in your hands to warm it up.) Always have an ample amount of this massage oil/lotion/hair conditioner nearby as well as small towels to wipe it off of your hands and her breasts after the massage is over.

Put a sizeable glob of massage oil/lotion/conditioner on each of your hands, rubbing it all over the palms of your hands to spread it out, as well as warm it if it's not yet warm. Then put your well lubricated hands on her breasts, *but not yet on her nipples and areolas*. This is because those provide the most pleasure and thus the best is saved for last!

It is so important that the massager make sure to keep his/her massaging hands *very* well lubricated. When the oil or lotion is breaking down the massager will feel stickiness developing. **It is now time to put more massage oil/lotion/conditioner on!** The rule of thumb is that you can't lubricate your hands and her breasts too much!

Also the massager needs to make sure his/her nails and skin of their hands are smooth. Trim and file your fingernails and that kind of thing, to as short and smooth as possible. Otherwise she (the person receiving the massage) might feel them as they rub against her sensitive skin. She can even get hurt by them because as she is in the thongs of ecstasy, she might not realize that they are hurting her, so make sure to watch out for her and take care of this situation.

Typically the massage will provide three levels of pleasure. Massaging the fleshy part of her breast (but not massaging her areolas and nipples) should give her pronounced and very welcome pleasure; of course the faster her breasts are massaged the more pleasure she'll get.

Including her areolas in the massaging will increase her pleasure a lot. But massaging her nipples will really get her going.

Below (and not in order of importance) are suggestions on how to optimize the breast massage.

* Start from the bottom of her breasts (where the breasts meet her torso) and work your way slowly higher up to just below her areolas. You can move your hands at varying speeds but typically the faster you massage the more pleasure she'll get.

* Simultaneously circle her boobs with each hand. Start out by using limited pressure on the breasts while utilizing only one finger, then gradually work your way up to utilizing all your fingers. Go clockwise then counterclockwise (or vice-versa.) Remember, *leave her nipples and areolas alone as much as possible until she's practically (or literally) begging for you to massage them.* Sure you will "bump" into them from time to time as you massage around them. Those bumps will give her a delicious taste of what's to come.

* At its base, wrap each hand around a single breast then run your well lubricated hands around and along that breast in a steady spiraling motion up the breasts in the direction of her nipples, until you reach the edge of her areolas. Of course you can go in the opposite direction also (starting from just below her areolas and working your way down to where her boobs meets her torso.)

* Place one hand on the base of one breast; the back of the hand should be facing her head. Put your other hand on the base of her *other* breast, the back of it should be facing her legs. Slide your well lubricated hands from left to right and then vice-versa, across and along both breasts.

* At its base, take each breast in a well lubricated hand and with increasing speed pull up from the base of her breast toward the nipple until your fingers reach the edge of the areolas (or if you're already playing with her areolas and/or nipples, go all the way to her nipples.) Then do the opposite and slide your hands back down

from the top of her breasts to the breast's base (where you started from.) Repeat this procedure many, many times.

* Tease her by sliding only your well lubricated, manicured fingertips over her breasts, wiggling your fingers.

* Instead of the above, perhaps for a minute or more, you'd like to start the festivities by teasing her breasts by only briefly touching them here and there using only the tips of your fingers.

* Concentrate your efforts on only one well lubricated breast; wrap both hands around it, kneading it, pulling it and twisting it.

As previously discussed, it's strongly suggested that you take your time before playing with her areolas and then nipples. This is because she will still get a good deal of pleasure from having the 'areola and nipple-less' massage. I for one require that she even beg you to play with her nipples--because as we know this is where the breasts offer the most pleasure.

Before finally massaging her nipples (admittedly you will "bump" into them periodically,) I would suggest waiting until she is already well stimulated. You may stroke her anticipation by whispering in her ear that you're about to play with her nipples, then suddenly do it! She may scream with delight as an orgasm overcomes her.

Playing with her nipples is typically the high point of the massage. She'll likely be getting the most pleasure now. (Again, the faster your well-lubricated fingers move around her nipples, the more pleasure she's likely to get.)

Okay massagers you now have a choice, you can immediately start massaging her nipples fast and hard, driving her crazy, or start massaging them slowly, then progressively massaging them faster and faster until she screams in ecstasy. If you're going to massage them fast immediately, as is the first option, many women will start their orgasm then (if they haven't already.)

Don't forget you can let her use a vibrator on herself as you massage her and thus it's suggested you keep a vibrator within her arm's reach. Believe me she'll find it if it's there.

Because so often the woman you're massaging will get so aroused from all this, that with both hands she'll instinctively reach around her lower back to play with the massager's pubic area. She then will not have a free hand to use the vibrator on herself. (Of course both your hands are busy giving her Extreme Pleasure Breast Massage.) A way to counter this is to secure a vibrator with white medical tape (the type used to hold gauge and cotton to cuts etc.) over her most sexually sensitive pubic area. (Perhaps it would be helpful if she keeps her panties on for extra support.) If you do this, more women will orgasm while you are giving her Extreme Pleasure Breast Massage.

Remember guys her nipples can get tender after orgasm and need to be left alone for at least a bit of time.

As is obvious, ladies, you can give yourself Extreme Pleasure Breast Massage in the privacy of your own bedroom.

After the massage, ladies your breasts tend to become firmer for a while and often they'll feel quite good for hours.

The following is another way of giving this massage, (told from the perspective of the kinky dominant massager.)

I will tell you to stand up and we will go to the bed (if we're not already there.) I will set the bed up so I am sitting with my back against the headboard of the bed and you are laying in front of me face-down on cushions (on the bed) with your head positioned so you can easily suck on my penis and play with my scrotum.

Also I'll put a roughly 3' x 3' sheet of plastic under your upper body to keep the massage lotion/oil/hair conditioner from going on the bed covers.

Perhaps I will also tie your hands together and perhaps then also to the headboard. If I do that though I will make sure there is enough slack in the rope for your hands to still move freely around my penis and scrotum while you suck. If your hands are tied to the headboard, I will be sitting on the rope as my butt will be in-between your bound hands and the headboard which your hands are tied to.

Your breasts will now be positioned, thanks to these cushions, just above the ground. As you suck on my penis, I will generously lubricate (and keep lubricated,) your breasts with some brand of preferably non-desensitizing massaging medium. I will warm the lotion/oil/hair conditioner up ahead of time or rub it in my hands to warm it up, if warming is necessary. I will then massage your breasts. (Many lotions put desensitizers in them to dull the pain of dry skin. These can at least partially desensitize breasts thus cutting down on the breast's capacity to provide pleasure.) I will continue for a long time to massage your lubricated breasts as you suck on my penis. (Remember to always keep the massager's hands well lubricated! The two of you will quickly notice that the nipples respond with the most pleasure from this massage.)

Using a yardstick type implement, I can reach across your back and spank you as you suck. Obviously one should make sure the woman can handle being spanked while sucking. Most can, depending on the intensity of the spanking and how hard she's already orgasming.

The End

www.ingramcontent.com/pod-product-compliance
Lightning Source LLC
Chambersburg PA
CBHW070606290526
45790CB00002B/806